Ehrlichiosis Disease Cookbook for Beginners

Balancing Your Diet for Optimal Health

Rhonda C Anderson MS RDN

mechanical methods, without the publisher's prior written permission.

Legal notice: This book is copyright protected; it can only be used for personal use. Without the publisher's or author's permission, you are not allowed to change, distribute, sell, quote from, or paraphrase any part of the book's contents.

Table of Contents

<u>Disclaimer</u>

We understand that living with Ehrlichiosis can be challenging and at times overwhelming.This cookbook is designed with love and care to help you navigate the dietary needs and lifestyle adjustments that come with managing this disease.

However, please remember that every person's journey with Ehrlichiosis is unique.The recipes and suggestions here are not a substitute for professional medical advice, diagnosis, or treatment. Always consult with your healthcare provider before making any significant changes to your diet or routine.

Our hearts are with you as you take each step toward wellness. We're here to support and encourage you, but your health and safety come first. Please prioritise the guidance of your medical team above all else.

Dedication

This cookbook is dedicated to you, the incredible souls who face each day with unwavering strength and courage. You navigate through challenges with bravery that inspires us all. Your journey is a testament to the human spirit's remarkable capacity for endurance and hope.

You are not alone. Though the path may be steep and the nights long, remember that your struggle does not go unnoticed. Each small victory, every moment of perseverance, is a beacon of hope and a story of triumph.

May this book be a companion on your journey, offering nourishment not just for your body, but also for your spirit. As you cook and create, know that you are cherished and admired for your extraordinary resilience.

With deepest admiration and support,

[RHONDA C ANDERSON MS RDN].

INTRODUCTION

*P*eter Leonard had always been a man full of life.

An avid hiker and nature enthusiast, he cherished his weekend adventures in the great outdoors. But one spring morning, everything changed.

After returning from a particularly strenuous hike, Peter noticed unusual symptoms: fever, muscle aches, and an overwhelming sense of fatigue.

What started as mild discomfort quickly escalated into a relentless battle against a mysterious illness. Doctors struggled to pinpoint the cause, until finally, Peter received a diagnosis—Ehrlichiosis Disease.

Ehrlichiosis, a tick-borne illness, had turned Peter's world upside down. The persistent symptoms drained his energy, and the treatments seemed to offer little respite.

Traditional medication left him feeling defeated and yearning for a more holistic approach. It was during this search for alternative solutions that Peter stumbled upon a transformative idea: could his diet hold the key to alleviating his suffering?

Determined to reclaim his health, Peter dove into research. He discovered that certain foods could bolster his immune system, reduce inflammation, and help his body combat the effects of Ehrlichiosis.

He meticulously crafted meals that not only nourished his body but also provided the necessary nutrients to aid in his recovery. With each carefully planned dish, Peter felt a resurgence of vitality. His symptoms gradually subsided, and he began to feel like himself again.

This is where "Ehrlichiosis Disease Cookbook for Beginners" by Rhonda C. Anderson steps in. Inspired by stories like Peter's, this cookbook is designed to be your guiding light on a journey to better health.

Inside these pages, you'll find more than just recipes; you'll discover a comprehensive approach to managing Ehrlichiosis through the power of food. Whether you're newly diagnosed or have been battling the disease for years, this book offers a lifeline—a way to take control of your health with every meal.

Our community of readers stands as a testament to the efficacy of these dietary strategies. In our private support group, 98% of our customers have reported significant improvements in their well-being after following the guidelines and recipes in our books.

These individuals, once grappling with the debilitating effects of Ehrlichiosis, now express true happiness and share remarkable stories of recovery. They've found a path to healing, and you can too.

By committing to the step-by-step instructions and embracing the nourishing recipes in this book, you too can join the ranks of those who have transformed their lives. "Ehrlichiosis Disease

Cookbook for Beginners" isn't just a collection of recipes—it's a roadmap to reclaiming your health and finding joy again. Dive in, follow along, and let the healing journey begin.

CHAPTER1:Understanding Ehrlichiosis and Its Dietary Impact.

1.1 What is Ehrlichiosis?

Ehrlichiosis is a bacterial infection transmitted to humans primarily through tick bites. The disease is caused by various species of the genus Ehrlichia, with Ehrlichia chaffeensis and Ehrlichia ewingii being the most common pathogens affecting humans.

1.2   Symptoms   and   Health Implications

1.Fever: This is usually the first symptom to appear and can be quite high, often exceeding 102°F (39°C).

2.Chills: Many people with ehrlichiosis experience chills along with their fever.

3.Severe Headache: A persistent and severe headache is a common symptom.

4.Muscle Aches (Myalgia): Muscle pain and general body aches are often reported.

5.Fatigue: There is often a profound sense of tiredness or weakness.

6.Nausea and Vomiting: Some people may experience gastrointestinal symptoms like nausea, vomiting, or diarrhoea.

7.Confusion or Brain Fog: In more severe cases, individuals might experience confusion or difficulty concentrating.

8.Rash: Although less common, some patients develop a rash. This is more frequently observed in children.

9.Joint Pain: Joint aches can also occur, adding to the general feeling of discomfort.

<u>Advanced Symptoms and Complications</u>

If ehrlichiosis is not treated promptly, it can lead to more severe symptoms and complications. These can include:

1.Respiratory Issues: In severe cases, individuals may experience breathing difficulties, including pneumonia.

2.Bleeding Problems: The infection can interfere with blood clotting, leading to unexplained bruising or bleeding.

3.Kidney and Liver Damage: Ehrlichiosis can affect these vital organs, potentially leading to liver function abnormalities or kidney failure.

4.Central Nervous System Involvement: Severe cases may involve the brain and spinal cord, leading to meningitis or encephalitis, causing severe headaches, neck stiffness, or even seizures.

5.Low Blood Cell Counts: The bacteria can attack and reduce the number of certain blood cells, leading to conditions like anaemia, leukopenia (low white blood cell count), or thrombocytopenia (low platelet count).

Diagnosis and Treatment

Diagnosing ehrlichiosis can be challenging due to the non-specific nature of its symptoms. Doctors typically rely on a combination of clinical signs, patient history (especially tick exposure), and laboratory tests. Blood tests can detect the presence of Ehrlichia bacteria or identify antibodies that the body produces in response to the infection.

The good news is that ehrlichiosis is treatable with antibiotics. Doxycycline is the antibiotic of choice and is most effective when started early in the course of the illness. It is usually given for 7 to 14 days. Prompt treatment is crucial as it can prevent complications and speed up recovery.

1.3 The Role of Diet in Managing Ehrlichiosis

Diet can significantly influence how your body copes with ehrlichiosis.

Here's how different types of foods can help:

1.Boosting Immunity with Nutrient-Rich Foods

Your immune system needs the right nutrients to function effectively. Foods high in vitamins, minerals, and antioxidants can help your body fight off the bacteria causing ehrlichiosis.

Key nutrients include:

Vitamin C: Found in citrus fruits, strawberries, and bell peppers, this vitamin boosts your immune response.

Zinc: Present in meats, nuts, and seeds, zinc helps with cell repair and immune function.

Vitamin E: Found in nuts and green leafy vegetables, vitamin E acts as an antioxidant, protecting your cells from damage.

Staying Hydrated

Fever and sweating can lead to dehydration, which can worsen your symptoms. Drinking plenty of fluids is crucial. Water is the best choice, but herbal teas and clear broths can also keep you hydrated. These fluids not only replace lost fluids but can also soothe your throat and provide comfort.

3.Eating Easy-to-Digest Foods

Ehrlichiosis can cause nausea and digestive upset. When your stomach is feeling unsettled, opt for foods that are gentle on your digestive system:

Bananas: Easy to digest and rich in potassium.
Rice: Provides energy without being heavy on your stomach.

Applesauce: Soft and easy on your digestive tract.
Toast: Simple and bland, helping to settle your stomach.

4.Avoiding Inflammatory Foods

Certain foods can increase inflammation in your body, which can make you feel worse. Try to avoid or limit:

Processed foods: These are often high in unhealthy fats and sugars.

Sugary drinks: They can lead to energy crashes and increased inflammation.
Alcohol: It can interfere with your immune system and hydration levels.

Chapter 2: Building a Nutrient-Rich Pantry

2.1 Essential Ingredients for Ehrlichiosis Diets

When dealing with ehrlichiosis, a balanced diet can support your recovery. Focus on these key ingredients:

1.Lean Proteins: Choose chicken, turkey, fish, and eggs for their easy-to-digest, muscle-repairing properties.

2.Fresh Vegetables: Incorporate leafy greens, bell peppers, broccoli, and Brussels sprouts for their vitamins and antioxidants.

3.Whole Grains: Opt for oats, quinoa, and brown rice to provide energy and aid digestion.

4.*Fruits:* Eat berries, citrus fruits, and bananas to boost immunity and energy levels.

5.*Healthy Fats:* Include avocados, nuts, seeds, and olive oil to support brain health and reduce inflammation.

6.*Herbs and Spices:* Use garlic, turmeric, and ginger for their immune-boosting and anti-inflammatory benefits.

7.*Hydration:* Stay hydrated with water, herbal teas, and nutrient-rich broths and soups.

2.2 Stocking Up on Anti-Inflammatory Foods

When it comes to ehrlichiosis, a tick-borne illness that causes flu-like symptoms, managing inflammation is crucial. Inflammation is the body's natural response to infection, but when it becomes excessive, it can lead to more discomfort and slow down recovery. That's where anti-inflammatory foods come into play. As a chef, I believe in the power of food not just to nourish, but also to heal. Let's explore some fantastic options to stock up on.

1. Leafy Greens

Start with leafy greens like spinach, kale, and Swiss chard. These vegetables are packed with vitamins and antioxidants that can help reduce inflammation. Spinach, for example, is rich in vitamin K, which helps curb inflammatory responses in the body. I love adding fresh spinach to salads or smoothies for a nutritious boost. Kale chips make for a delightful, crispy snack.

2. Berries

Berries such as blueberries, strawberries, and raspberries are small but mighty when it comes to their anti-inflammatory properties. These fruits are loaded with antioxidants called flavonoids, which can help combat inflammation. A berry parfait with yogurt and honey is a delicious and refreshing way to enjoy these fruits. You can also toss them into a morning bowl of oatmeal for a colorful start to your day.

3.Fatty Fish

Salmon, mackerel, and sardines are excellent sources of omega-3 fatty acids. Omega-3s are renowned for their ability to reduce inflammation. Grilled salmon with a side of roasted vegetables not only makes a tasty meal but also supports your body's fight against inflammation. If you're not a fan of fish, omega-3 supplements can be a good alternative, but always consult with a healthcare professional first.

4.Nuts and Seeds

Walnuts, almonds, chia seeds, and flaxseeds are rich in healthy fats and fiber, both of which help reduce inflammation. A handful of nuts makes a great snack, or you can sprinkle seeds over your salads and cereals. I often use ground flaxseeds in my baking for an added health kick. Chia seeds soaked in almond milk with a touch of honey make a wonderful pudding.

5.Olive Oil

Olive oil is a staple in Mediterranean cuisine, and for good reason. It's packed with monounsaturated fats and antioxidants, especially oleocanthal, which acts similarly to anti-inflammatory drugs. Use extra-virgin olive oil for dressings, drizzling over roasted vegetables, or in cooking to reap its full benefits. A simple caprese salad with tomatoes, mozzarella, basil, and a drizzle of olive oil is both elegant and anti-inflammatory.

6.Turmeric

Turmeric is a vibrant yellow spice known for its powerful anti-inflammatory properties, largely due to its active ingredient, curcumin. Incorporate turmeric into your cooking with dishes like curries or sprinkle it over roasted vegetables. Turmeric tea, made with warm milk and a pinch of black pepper, is a soothing drink that helps your body absorb curcumin more effectively.

7.Garlic and Ginger

Both garlic and ginger have strong anti-inflammatory effects and are commonly used in cooking worldwide. Garlic can be added to nearly any savory dish to enhance flavor and health benefits. Ginger, with its warm, spicy kick, is fantastic in stir-fries, soups, and even desserts. Ginger tea, made with fresh ginger slices steeped in hot water, is perfect for calming an upset stomach and reducing inflammation.

8.Tomatoes

Tomatoes are rich in lycopene, an antioxidant that has been shown to reduce inflammation. Cooked tomatoes, like those in sauces and soups, have higher lycopene content than fresh ones. A hearty tomato soup or a homemade marinara sauce over whole-grain pasta is a comforting and nutritious way to include more tomatoes in your diet.

9.Green Tea

Green tea is packed with antioxidants called catechins, which help fight inflammation. Enjoying a cup of green tea daily can provide a gentle but steady anti-inflammatory effect. Matcha, a powdered form of green tea, can be added to smoothies, baked goods, or simply enjoyed as a frothy, warm beverage.

10. Dark Chocolate

Yes, chocolate can be part of an anti-inflammatory diet! Dark chocolate, with at least 70% cocoa content, contains flavonoids that reduce inflammation. Indulge in a small piece of dark chocolate as a treat or use it in baking for a rich,

satisfying flavour. Just remember, moderation is key

Chapter 3: Breakfast Boosters: Energise Your Morning

1.Overnight Oatmeal with Fresh Raspberries.

Prep Time:5 mins
Additional Time:8 hrs
Total Time:8 hrs 5 mins
Servings:1

Ingredients.
- ½ cup old-fashioned rolled oats
- ½ cup fat-free milk
- ¼ teaspoon ground cinnamon
- 1 pinch salt
- 1 teaspoon maple syrup
- ⅛ cup fresh raspberries

Directions.

1. In a small container, mix together oats, milk, cinnamon, salt, and maple syrup. Stir well, cover the container, and place it in the refrigerator overnight.
2. In the morning, add fresh raspberries on top before serving.

<u>Nutritional value</u>
Carbs:40g
Fat:3g
Calories:221
Protein:15g

2.Grilled Greek Yogurt Marinated Chicken

Prep Time:15 mins
Cook Time:35 mins
Additional Time:3 hrs
Total Time:3 hrs 50 mins
Servings:6

Ingredients.

- ½ cup plain low-fat Greek yoghourt
- 4 cloves garlic, crushed
- ½ lemon, juiced
- 1 tablespoon lemon zest
- 1 tablespoon olive oil
- 1 tablespoon paprika
- 1 teaspoon herbes de Provence
- 1 teaspoon salt
- 1 teaspoon ground black pepper
- 1 (5 pound) whole chicken, cut into 8 pieces
- 1 pinch salt

Yoghourt Sauce:

- ½ cup plain low-fat Greek yoghourt
- 1 tablespoon lemon juice
- 1 teaspoon harissa

Directions.

1. In a medium bowl, mix together the yoghurt, minced garlic, lemon juice and zest, olive oil, paprika, herbes de Provence, salt, and black pepper. Transfer this mixture to a large resealable plastic bag. Add the chicken pieces to the bag and ensure

they are well-coated with the marinade. Expel as much air as possible from the bag before sealing it. Refrigerate for a minimum of 3 hours to marinate.

2. Preheat your outdoor grill to medium-high heat and oil the grate lightly to prevent sticking.

3. To prepare the sauce, combine yoghurt, lemon juice, and harissa in a small bowl. Stir until smooth and set aside.

4. Remove the chicken from the marinade and place it on a plate or baking sheet lined with paper towels. Discard the used marinade. Pat the chicken pieces dry with additional paper towels and sprinkle with a little salt.

5. Grill the chicken with the skin-side down for 2 minutes on the preheated grill. Flip each piece and shift them to indirect heat. Continue grilling with the lid closed, turning the chicken often, until it is evenly browned and the internal temperature reaches 165°F (74°C), approximately 30 to 35 minutes.

6. Serve the grilled chicken with the prepared sauce on the side.

Nutritional value
Carbs:6g

Fat:30g
Calories:523
Protein:55g

3.Kale and Banana Smoothie

Prep Time:5 mins
Total Time:5 mins
Servings:1.

Ingredients.

- 2 cups chopped kale
- 1 banana
- ½ cup light unsweetened soy milk
- 1 tablespoon flax seeds
- 1 teaspoon maple syrup

Directions.

1. Collect all the ingredients.
2. Add kale, banana, soy milk, flax seeds, and maple syrup to the blender.
3. Blend until the mixture is smooth.
4. Pour over ice and serve.

<u>**Nutritional value**</u>
Carbs:59g
Fat:9g
Calories:311
Protein:12g

4.Scrambled Eggs, Cheese, and Avocado Tortilla Bowl.

Prep Time:10 mins
Cook Time:6 mins
Additional Time:2 mins
Total Time:18 mins
Servings:1

Ingredients.

- 1 (10 inch) soft flour tortilla
- 2 eggs
- ½ teaspoon milk
- ½ teaspoon butter (Optional)
- ¼ cup shredded Mexican cheese blend, or more to taste
- ½ avocado - peeled, pitted, and diced

- ¼ cup salsa, or to taste (Optional)
- 1 pinch paprika, or to taste (Optional)
- 1 pinch sea salt

Directions.

1. Heat your oven to 400°F (200°C). Shape the tortilla by pressing it into a tortilla shell mold or an oven-safe bowl.

2. In a microwave-safe bowl, whisk together the eggs, milk, and butter. Mix in the Mexican cheese blend.

3. Bake the tortilla in the oven until it's crispy and golden brown, approximately 5 to 7 minutes. Let it cool slightly, then carefully remove it from the mold and place it on a serving plate, about 2 minutes later.

4. Microwave the egg mixture until it begins to set, for 30 seconds to 1 minute. Stir gently with a fork and microwave again until fully set, another 30 seconds.

5. Fill the crispy tortilla bowl with the cooked eggs and garnish with avocado, salsa, paprika, and a pinch of salt.

Nutritional value
Carbs:51g
Fat:43g
Calories:690
Protein:29g

5.Eggnog French Toast

Prep Time:15 mins
Cook Time:10 mins
Total Time:25 mins
Servings:6

Ingredients.

- 1 ½ cups eggnog
- 2 large eggs, beaten slightly
- 1 ½ tablespoons ground cinnamon, or to taste
- 1 teaspoon pumpkin pie spice
- 12 slices French bread

Directions.

1. In a mixing bowl, combine eggnog, eggs, cinnamon, and pumpkin pie spice. Whisk the ingredients until they are thoroughly blended. Transfer the mixture to a shallow dish.

2. Set an electric skillet to 300 degrees F (150 degrees C) and lightly grease it.

3. One by one, dip each slice of bread into the eggnog mixture, ensuring that both sides are fully coated.

4. Arrange the coated bread slices on the preheated skillet and cook them, turning once, until both sides are golden brown. Place the cooked slices on a serving plate, cover with foil to keep them warm until all slices are ready. Serve immediately.

Nutritional value
Carbs:19g
Fat:9g
Calories:158
Protein:6g

6.Chia Seed Pudding:

Prep Time:15 mins
Additional Time:8 hrs 30 minutes
Total Time:8 hrs 45 mins
Servings:4

Ingredients.

- 1 cup unsweetened vanilla-flavoured almond milk
- 1 cup vanilla fat-free yoghourt
- 2 tablespoons pure maple syrup
- 1 teaspoon pure vanilla extract
- ⅛ teaspoon salt
- ¼ cup chia seeds
- 1 pint strawberries, hulled and chopped
- 4 teaspoons pure maple syrup
- ¼ cup toasted almonds

Directions.

1. In a bowl, combine the almond milk, yoghourt, 2 tablespoons of maple syrup, vanilla, and salt. Whisk until smooth. Stir in the chia seeds until they are evenly distributed and let the mixture sit for 30 minutes to allow the seeds to absorb the liquid.

2. After 30 minutes, stir the mixture to ensure the chia seeds are evenly mixed. Cover the bowl with plastic wrap and refrigerate for at least 8 hours or overnight.

3. In a separate bowl, coat the strawberries with 4 teaspoons of maple syrup and mix well. Add the almonds and stir to combine.

4. Serve the chia seed pudding in 4 bowls, and top each with the strawberry and almond mixture.

<u>Nutritional value</u>
Carbs:38g
Fat:8g
Calories:243
Protein:6g

7.Whipped Cottage Cheese

Prep Time:5 mins
Total Time:5 mins
Servings:6

Ingredients.

- 1 (16 ounce container) low-fat cottage cheese

<u>Sweet Option:</u>

- 2 tablespoons honey, or to taste

Directions.

1. Put the cottage cheese into the food processor or blender. Process for about a minute until smooth, pausing halfway through to scrape down the sides. If you prefer a sweeter taste, add honey and blend until you reach the desired level of sweetness.

<u>Nutritional value</u>
Carbs:8g
Fat:1g
Calories:76
Protein:11g

8.Asparagus Omelette

Prep Time:15 mins
Cook Time:30 mins

Total Time:45 mins
Servings:2

Ingredients.

- 6 strips bacon
- 10 stalks asparagus, trimmed
- 1 teaspoon vegetable oil, or as needed
- ⅓ red onion, diced
- ½ tomato, diced
- 3 button mushrooms, sliced
- 5 eggs
- 3 tablespoons heavy whipping cream
- 1 pinch freshly ground nutmeg
- salt and ground black pepper to taste
- ½ cup grated mozzarella cheese

Directions.

1. Place the bacon in a large skillet and cook it over medium-high heat, turning occasionally, until it is evenly browned, which will take about 10 minutes. Transfer the bacon slices to paper towels to drain. Once cooled, crumble the bacon into pieces.

2. Fill a large pot with lightly salted water and bring it to a boil. Add the asparagus and cook until it is tender but still firm, about 2 to 3 minutes. Drain and set aside.

3. In a skillet, heat the vegetable oil over medium-high heat. Sauté the onion, tomato, and mushrooms until they are tender, approximately 5 minutes.

4. In a bowl, whisk together the eggs and cream. Mix in the crumbled bacon, sautéed vegetables, asparagus, nutmeg, salt, and pepper.

5. Pour the egg mixture into an oven-safe nonstick skillet and cover. Cook over medium-low heat until the omelette is set, which should take about 10 to 12 minutes. Sprinkle mozzarella cheese on top.

6. Adjust the oven rack to about 6 inches from the broiler and preheat the broiler.

7. Place the skillet under the preheat broiler and broil the omelette until the top develops a golden crust, about 2 minutes.

<u>Nutritional value</u>
Carbs:12g
Fat:45g

Calories:546
Protein:42g

9.Whole Grain Pancakes:

Prep Time:15 mins
Cook Time:15 mins
Total Time:30 mins
Servings:4

Ingredients.

- 1 cup whole wheat flour
- ½ cup rolled oats
- ¼ cup cornmeal
- 3 tablespoons flaxseed meal
- 3 tablespoons brown sugar
- 1 teaspoon baking powder
- ½ teaspoon baking soda
- 1 egg, beaten
- 2 cups buttermilk
- cooking spray

Directions.

1. In a large mixing bowl, combine whole wheat flour, oats, cornmeal, flaxseed meal, brown sugar, baking powder, and baking soda. Add the buttermilk and egg, then stir until the mixture is smooth.

2. Preheat a large skillet or griddle over medium heat and lightly coat it with cooking spray. Spoon the batter onto the griddle in large dollops, cooking until bubbles appear and the edges begin to set. Flip the pancakes and cook until the other side is golden brown. Continue this process with the remaining batter.

<u>Nutritional value</u>
Carbs:57g
Fat:9g
Calories:308
Protein:13g

10.Blueberry Lemon Breakfast Quinoa.

Prep Time:5 mins

Cook Time:25 mins
Total Time:30 mins
Servings:2

Ingredients.

- 1 cup quinoa
- 2 cups nonfat milk
- 1 pinch salt
- 3 tablespoons maple syrup
- ½ lemon, zested
- 1 cup blueberries
- 2 teaspoons flax seed

Directions.

1. Thoroughly rinse the quinoa in a fine-mesh strainer under cold water until the water runs clear and any froth is gone, to eliminate bitterness.

2. In a saucepan, warm the milk over medium heat for 2 to 3 minutes. Add the rinsed quinoa and a pinch of salt to the milk, and let it simmer on medium-low heat for about 20 minutes, until most of the liquid is absorbed. Take the saucepan off the

heat and stir in the maple syrup and lemon zest. Gently incorporate the blueberries.

3. Divide the quinoa mixture into two bowls and sprinkle each serving with a teaspoon of flaxseed before serving.

<u>Nutritional value</u>
Carbs:99g
Fat:9g
Calories:542

Protein:24g

Chapter 4: Lunch Solutions: Delicious Midday Meals

1.Grilled Chicken Salad with Seasonal Fruit

Prep Time:15 mins
Cook Time:20 mins
Total Time:35 mins
Servings:6

Ingredients.

- 1 pound skinless, boneless chicken breast halves
- ½ cup pecans
- ⅓ cup red wine vinegar
- ½ cup white sugar
- 1 cup vegetable oil
- ½ onion, minced
- 1 teaspoon ground mustard
- 1 teaspoon salt

- ¼ teaspoon ground white pepper
- 2 heads Bibb lettuce - rinsed, dried and torn
- 1 cup sliced fresh strawberries

Directions.

1. Heat the grill on high and lightly grease the grill grate.

2. Cook the chicken on the grill until fully cooked, approximately 8 minutes per side. Remove from heat, let it cool, and then slice. Set aside.

3. In a skillet over medium-high heat, toast the pecans until they become fragrant, stirring often, for about 8 minutes. Remove from heat and set aside.

4. For the dressing: Blend red wine vinegar, sugar, vegetable oil, onion, mustard, salt, and pepper until smooth.

5. Place lettuce on plates. Top with sliced grilled chicken, strawberries, and toasted pecans. Drizzle with the dressing before serving.

<u>**Nutritional value**</u>
Carbs:23
Fat:48g
Calories:569
Protein:19g

2.Vegetable Soup

Prep Time:15 mins
Cook Time:35
Total Time:50 mins
Servings:6

Ingredients.

- 1 (14.5 ounce) can diced tomatoes
- 1 (14 ounce) can chicken broth
- 1 (11.5 ounce) can tomato-vegetable juice cocktail
- 2 carrots, sliced
- 2 stalks celery, diced
- 1 large potato, diced
- 1 cup chopped fresh green beans
- 1 cup fresh corn kernels
- 1 cup water

- salt and pepper to taste
- 1 pinch Creole seasoning, or more to taste

Directions.

1. Collect all the ingredients needed.

2. Mix together tomatoes, chicken broth, tomato juice, carrots, celery, potato, green beans, corn, and water in a large soup pot. Season with salt, pepper, and Creole seasoning.

3. Heat the mixture until it boils, then reduce the heat and let it simmer until the vegetables are soft, which usually takes about 30 minutes.

4. Serve the soup hot and enjoy your meal!

<u>Nutritional value</u>
Carbs:24g
Fat:1
Calories:116
Protein:4g

3.Quinoa Patties

Prep Time:15 mins
Cook Time:25 mins
Total Time:40 mins
Servings:14.

Ingredients.

- 1 cup low-sodium vegetable broth
- 1 cup dry quinoa, rinsed and drained
- ¾ cup water
- 3 tablespoons olive oil, or more as needed, divided
- 1 white onion, chopped
- 1 zucchini, grated
- 1 large carrot, grated
- garlic powder, or more to taste
- salt and ground black pepper to taste
- 4 large eggs, lightly beaten
- ½ cup oat groats, ground into a powder

Directions.

1. Combine vegetable broth, water, and quinoa in a saucepan. Bring to a boil, then lower the heat. Cover and simmer until quinoa is tender and liquid is absorbed, about 15 to 20 minutes. Spread cooked quinoa on a large platter to cool.

2. Heat 1 tablespoon of olive oil in a large skillet over medium heat. Sauté onion, zucchini, and carrot until onion turns translucent, about 3 to 5 minutes. Transfer vegetables to a plate and let them cool.

3. In a large bowl, mix the cooled vegetables with 3 cups of the cooled quinoa. Season with garlic powder, salt, and black pepper. Add eggs and ground oats, stirring until well combined. Divide the mixture into 14 portions and shape into patties.

4. Heat 2 tablespoons of olive oil in a large skillet over medium heat. Fry the patties until browned, approximately 2 minutes per side. Add more oil as needed between batches.

Nutritional value
Carbs:14g

Fat:5g
Calories:120
Protein:5g

4.Honey Coconut Salmon

Prep Time:15 mins
Cook Time:35 mins
Additional Time:30 mins
Total Time:1 hr 20 mins
Servings:4

Ingredients.

- 1 ½ cups butter
- ¾ cup honey
- ¼ cup brown sugar
- ¾ cup flaked coconut
- 4 (4 ounce) fillets salmon

Directions.

1. Heat butter in a saucepan over medium heat. Add honey, brown sugar, and coconut. Bring to a boil, then remove from heat. Let cool slightly, then

transfer to a large bowl. Place salmon in the bowl, coat with the mixture, cover, and marinate in the refrigerator for at least 30 minutes.

2. Preheat the oven to 375°F (190°C).

3. Spread a portion of the marinade in a baking dish to coat the bottom. Arrange salmon in the dish and pour some marinade over the top, ensuring coconut is evenly distributed.

4. Bake for 25 minutes in the preheated oven, occasionally basting with the remaining marinade, until the salmon flakes easily with a fork. Discard any extra marinade or boil it for 5 minutes, then spoon over the salmon before serving.

<u>Nutritional value</u>
Carbs:12g
Fat:16g
Calories:215
Protein:12g

5. Turkey Avocado Panini

Prep Time:17 mins
Cook Time:8 mins
Total Time:25 mins
Servings:2

Ingredients.

- ½ ripe avocado
- ¼ cup mayonnaise
- 2 ciabatta rolls
- 1 tablespoon olive oil, divided
- 2 slices provolone cheese
- 1 cup whole fresh spinach leaves, divided
- ¼ pound thinly sliced mesquite smoked turkey breast
- 2 roasted red peppers, sliced into strips

Directions.

1. Combine mashed avocado and mayonnaise in a bowl until well blended.

2. Preheat a panini press.

3. To assemble the sandwiches, cut the ciabatta rolls horizontally and brush the bottom halves with olive oil. Place the bottoms on the panini press, olive oil side down. Layer provolone cheese, spinach leaves, turkey breast slices, and roasted red pepper slices on each sandwich. Spread avocado mixture on the cut side of the top halves and place them on the sandwiches. Brush the top of each roll with olive oil.

4. Close the panini press and cook until the rolls are toasted with golden brown grill marks and the cheese is melted, approximately 5 to 8 minutes.

Nutritional value
Carbs:42g
Fat:53g
Calories:724
Protein:25g

6. Tasty Egg Salad

Prep Time:10 mins
Cook Time:15 mins
Additional Time:10 mins
Total Time:35 mins
Servings:4

Ingredients.

- 8 large eggs
- ½ cup mayonnaise
- ¼ cup chopped green onion
- 1 teaspoon prepared yellow mustard
- ¼ teaspoon paprika
- salt and pepper to taste

Directions.

1. Put the eggs into a saucepan and cover them with cold water. Bring the water to a boil, then take the saucepan off the heat. Let the eggs sit in the hot water, covered, for 10 to 12 minutes. Remove the eggs from the hot water, cool them down, peel off the shells, and chop them.

2. Place the chopped eggs into a bowl. Mix in mayonnaise, green onion, and mustard. Season with paprika, salt, and pepper. Stir well. Serve the mixture on your preferred choice of bread, crackers, or salad greens.

Nutritional value
Carbs:2g
Fat:30g
Calories:333
Protein:13g

7.White Bean Chicken Breast Chili

Prep Time:20 mins
Cook Time:30 mins
Total Time:50 mins
Servings:4

Ingredients.
- 1 teaspoon vegetable oil
- 2 boneless, skinless chicken breast halves

- 1 teaspoon vegetable oil
- 1 large onion, diced
- salt and freshly ground black pepper to taste
- 4 cloves garlic, chopped
- 1 tablespoon ancho chile powder
- 1 teaspoon ground cumin
- 1 teaspoon all-purpose flour
- ½ teaspoon chipotle pepper powder
- ¼ teaspoon dried oregano
- 1 teaspoon fine cornmeal
- 2 cups chicken broth, divided
- 2 (15 ounce) cans white beans, drained
- 1 cup chicken broth
- ¼ teaspoon white sugar, or to taste
- 1 pinch cayenne pepper, or to taste
- ⅓ cup chopped green onions
- ⅓ cup sour cream
- ⅓ cup chopped fresh cilantro

Directions.

1. Heat 1 teaspoon of vegetable oil in a large, deep skillet over medium-high heat. Cook the chicken breasts until they are browned, approximately 4 minutes per side. Reduce the heat to medium, flip

the breasts, cover the pan, and continue cooking until the other side is browned, about 5 minutes more. Transfer the chicken to a plate and let it cool before chopping it into cubes.

2. Return the skillet to medium heat, add another teaspoon of vegetable oil, along with onion, salt, and black pepper. Cook and stir until the onion becomes translucent, which should take about 4 to 5 minutes. Add the garlic and cook for another minute until fragrant.

3. Stir in ancho chilli powder, cumin, flour, chipotle pepper powder, and oregano into the onion mixture. Cook and stir for 2 to 3 minutes until fragrant. Pour in 1 cup of chicken broth, stirring to scrape up any browned bits from the bottom of the pan. Add cornmeal and bring the mixture to a simmer.

4. Stir in beans and another cup of chicken broth. Cut the cooled chicken breasts into cubes and add them to the chilli mixture. Bring everything to a simmer. Pour in the remaining cup of chicken

broth, season with salt, black pepper, sugar, and cayenne pepper according to your taste. Cook until everything is heated through. Serve the chilli garnished with green onions, sour cream, and cilantro.

<u>Nutritional value</u>
Carbs:55g
Fat:12g
Calories:410
Protein:32g

8.Miso Soup

Prep Time:5 mins
Cook Time:10 mins
Total Time:15 mins
Servings:4

Ingredients.
- 4 cups water
- 2 teaspoons dashi granules
- 3 tablespoons miso paste

- 1 (8 ounce) package silken tofu, diced
- 2 green onions, sliced diagonally into 1/2 inch pieces

Directions.

1. In a medium saucepan, bring water and dashi granules to a boil over medium-high heat. Reduce to medium heat and whisk in miso paste. Add tofu and gently simmer for 2 to 3 minutes. Separate green onion layers and add to the soup before serving.

Nutritional value
Carbs:5g
Fat:2g
Calories:67
Protein:7g

9.Perfect Ten Baked Cod:

Prep Time:10 mins

Cook Time:25 mins
Total Time:35 mins
Servings:4

Ingredients.

- 4 tablespoons butter, divided
- ½ sleeve buttery round crackers (such as Ritz®), crushed
- 1 pound thick-cut cod loin
- ½ medium lemon, juiced
- ¼ cup dry white wine
- 1 tablespoon chopped fresh parsley
- 1 tablespoon chopped green onion
- 1 medium lemon, cut into wedges

Directions.

1. Prepare all ingredients.

2. Preheat the oven to 400°F (200°C).

3. Put 2 tablespoons of butter in a microwave-safe bowl and melt it in the microwave for about 30 seconds. Mix in the crushed butter crackers.

4. Place the remaining 2 tablespoons of butter in a 7x11-inch baking dish and melt it in the preheated

oven for 1 to 3 minutes. Remove the dish from the oven.

5. Coat both sides of the cod with the melted butter in the baking dish.

6. Bake the cod in the preheated oven for 10 minutes. Take it out, sprinkle it with lemon juice, wine, and the cracker mixture. Return to the oven and bake until the fish is opaque and flakes easily with a fork, about another 10 minutes.

7. Garnish with parsley and green onion. Serve with lemon wedges.

<u>Nutritional value</u>
Carbs:21g
Fat:17g
Calories:280
Protein:23v

10.Greek Yogurt Breakfast Parfait

Prep Time:10 mins
Total Time:10 mins
Servings:2

Ingredients.

- ½ cup fresh blueberries
- ½ cup sliced fresh strawberries
- 1 teaspoon white sugar (Optional)
- 6 tablespoons granola, or as needed
- 1 (6 ounce) container nonfat vanilla Greek yoghourt
- 1 teaspoon lemon zest

Directions.

1. Combine blueberries and strawberries in a small bowl. Mix with sugar until the berries are coated.

2. In each of 2 parfait glasses, start with a layer of 2 tablespoons of granola. Add 2 tablespoons of yoghourt on top, sprinkling with 1/2 teaspoon of lemon zest. Follow with a third of the berry mixture. Repeat these layers until the glasses are filled.

Nutritional value
Carbs:27g
Fat:14g
Calories:265

**Protein:12g

Chapter 5: Satisfying Dinners: Balanced Evening Meals

1.Grilled Masala Chicken with Vegetables

Prep Time:25 mins
Cook Time:25 mins
Total Time:50 mins
Servings:4

Ingredients.

- ¼ cup olive oil
- 6 teaspoons garam masala, divided
- 4 small cloves garlic, minced
- 1 teaspoon salt
- ½ teaspoon ground black pepper
- Reynolds Wrap® Heavy Duty Aluminum Foil

- 4 (5 ounce) skinless, boneless chicken breast halves
- 4 small yellow summer squash or zucchini, sliced into 1/4-inch rounds
- 1 medium sweet onion, thinly sliced
- ½ cup plain yoghourt
- 1 teaspoon Cilantro leaves

Directions.

1. Combine olive oil, 4 teaspoons of garam masala, minced garlic, salt, and black pepper in a small bowl. Mix until well blended.

2. Tear four sheets of Reynolds Wrap® Heavy Duty Aluminum Foil, each measuring 12x18 inches. Place one chicken breast half in the centre of each sheet. Sprinkle both sides of the chicken with 1/2 teaspoon of garam masala.

3. Arrange squash and onion slices on top of each chicken breast. Drizzle evenly with one-fourth of the olive oil mixture. Fold up the sides of the foil to create packets, folding the top and ends twice to seal

tightly while leaving space for heat circulation. Repeat for the remaining packets.

4. Grill the foil packets over medium-high heat with the grill covered for 20 to 25 minutes, or until the chicken is thoroughly cooked (internal temperature of 165 degrees F).

5. Carefully open the packets by cutting along the top fold with a sharp knife to release steam, then unfold the top of the foil packet. Serve topped with yoghourt and optionally garnish with cilantro.

Nutritional value
Carbs:15g
Fat:18g
Calories:357
Protein:41g

2.Hot Spinach Artichoke Dip

Prep Time:15 mins
Cook Time:25 mins
Total Time:40 mins
Servings:12

Ingredients.

- 1 (8 ounce) package cream cheese, softened
- ¼ cup mayonnaise
- ¼ cup grated Parmesan cheese
- ¼ cup grated Romano cheese
- 1 clove garlic, peeled and minced
- ½ teaspoon dried basil
- ¼ teaspoon garlic salt
- salt and pepper to taste
- 1 (14 ounce) can artichoke hearts, drained and chopped
- ½ cup frozen chopped spinach, thawed and drained
- ¼ cup shredded mozzarella cheese

Directions.

1. Preheat your oven to 350 degrees Fahrenheit (175 degrees Celsius) and lightly grease a small baking dish.

2. In a medium bowl, combine cream cheese, mayonnaise, Parmesan cheese, Romano cheese, garlic, basil, garlic salt, salt, and pepper. Add in artichoke hearts and spinach, gently mixing everything together.

3.Transfer the mixture into the prepared baking dish and sprinkle mozzarella cheese on top. Bake in the preheated oven until the dish is bubbly and lightly browned, which should take about 25 minutes.

<u>Nutritional value</u>
Carbs:3g
Fat:12g
Calories:134
Protein:4g

3.Black Bean Vegetable Soup

Prep Time:15 mins
Cook Time:20 mins
Total Time:35 mins
Servings:8

Ingredients.
- 1 tablespoon vegetable oil
- 4 carrots, chopped
- 1 onion, chopped
- 4 cloves garlic, minced

- 1 tablespoon chilli powder
- 1 teaspoon ground cumin
- 4 cups chicken broth
- 3 (15 ounce) cans black beans, rinsed and drained, divided

Directions.

1. Heat oil in a large saucepan over medium heat. Sauté carrots, onion, and garlic until the onion softens, about 5 minutes. Add chilli powder and cumin, and cook until evenly coated, about 2 minutes.

2. Pour broth into the saucepan with the onion mixture. Add half of the black beans, corn, and black pepper. Bring to a boil.

3. Blend tomatoes and the remaining black beans until smooth using a food processor or blender. Add this mixture to the broth. Reduce heat to low, cover, and simmer until carrots are tender, approximately 10 to 15 minutes.

<u>Nutritional value</u>
Carbs:42g
Fat:3g

Calories:238
Protein:12g

4.Broccoli Rice Casserole

Prep Time:10 mins
Cook Time:35 mins
Total Time:45 mins
Servings:10

Ingredients.

- 2 (10 ounce) packages frozen chopped broccoli
- 2 tablespoons butter, divided
- 1 cup celery, chopped
- 1 cup onion, chopped
- 2 clove garlic, minced
- 1 (10.5 ounce) can condensed cream of mushroom soup
- 1 (10.5 ounce) can condensed cream of chicken soup
- 2/3 cup milk
- 8 ounces Muenster or Swiss cheese, shredded
- 2 teaspoons Dijon mustard

- 1/2 teaspoon paprika
- 1/2 teaspoon freshly ground black pepper
- 3 cups cooked long grain white rice
- 1/2 cup panko bread crumbs

Directions.

1. Gather all the necessary ingredients. Preheat your oven to 350°F (175°C) and grease a 3-quart baking dish.

2. Place the broccoli and 2 tablespoons of water in a large microwave-safe bowl. Cover it with plastic wrap and microwave on high for 5 minutes, stirring once. Drain the broccoli.

3. In a large skillet over medium heat, melt 1 tablespoon of butter. Add celery, onion, and garlic. Cook and stir until tender, approximately 3 to 5 minutes.

4. Add the soup and milk to the skillet. Heat the mixture until warmed through.

5. Combine the cooked vegetable mixture with the broccoli in the microwave-safe bowl.

6. Mix in shredded cheese, mustard, paprika, and pepper.

7. Stir in the rice until everything is well combined. Spoon the mixture into the greased baking dish.

8. Transfer the mixture into the prepared baking dish. Combine the panko with the remaining 1 tablespoon of melted butter. Sprinkle this mixture on top of the casserole.

9. Bake in the preheated oven until the top is golden brown and the casserole is bubbly, which usually takes about 30 to 40 minutes.

10. Serve and enjoy your delicious casserole!

<u>Nutritional value</u>
Carbs:31g
Fat:14g
Calories:297
Protein:12g

5.Whole Grain Healthy Banana Bread

Prep Time:15 mins
Cook Time:1 hr
Total Time:1 hr 15 mins
Servings:10

Ingredients.

- ¾ cup SPLENDA® Sugar Blend
- ¾ cup flaxseed meal
- 5 ripe bananas, mashed
- ¼ cup skim milk
- ¼ cup low-fat sour cream
- 2 teaspoons egg whites
- 2 cups whole wheat flour
- 1 teaspoon baking soda
- ½ teaspoon salt

Directions.

1. Preheat your oven to 350 degrees Fahrenheit (175 degrees Celsius) and grease a 9x5 inch loaf pan.

2. In a medium bowl, thoroughly combine the sugar substitute, ground flaxseed, bananas, milk, sour cream, and egg whites. In a separate bowl, mix the flour, baking soda, and salt, then add it to the banana mixture, stirring until just combined. Transfer the batter into the greased loaf pan.

3. Bake in the preheated oven for about 1 hour and 10 minutes, or until a toothpick inserted into the centre of the loaf comes out clean.

<u>**Nutritional value**</u>
Carbs:48g
Fat:5g
Calories:262
Protein:6g

6.Summer Grilled Shrimp Salad

Prep Time:30 mins
Cook Time:5 mins
Total Time:35 mins
Servings:2

Ingredients.

- 1 tablespoon olive oil
- 2 ¼ teaspoons smokehouse maple seasoning (such as McCormick Grill Mates)
- 1 ½ teaspoons lemon juice
- 12 ounces peeled and deveined shrimp

<u>Cilantro Vinaigrette:</u>

- ¼ cup extra-virgin olive oil

- 2 tablespoons honey
- 2 tablespoons fresh lime juice
- 2 tablespoons chopped cilantro
- 1 tablespoon balsamic vinegar
- salt and ground black pepper to taste

Salad:
- 4 cups mixed salad greens, or more to taste
- ½ cup thinly sliced English cucumber
- ⅓ cup freshly cooked corn
- ½ cup diced tomato
- ¼ cup sliced red onion
- 1 avocado, diced

Directions.

1. Combine olive oil, maple seasoning, and lemon juice in a glass bowl. Mix well with shrimp until coated. Chill in the refrigerator until ready to grill.

2. In a small bowl, whisk together olive oil, honey, lime juice, cilantro, balsamic vinegar, salt, and pepper to make the vinaigrette. Set aside.

3. Heat an indoor or outdoor grill to medium-high. Skewer the shrimp and grill until they turn pink

and opaque, approximately 2 minutes per side. Remove from skewers and set aside.

4. Arrange mixed greens in a large salad bowl. Arrange cucumber, corn, tomato, red onion, and avocado in sections over the greens. Place the grilled shrimp in the centre. Drizzle with vinaigrette, toss gently to coat, and serve immediately.

<u>Nutritional value</u>
Carbs:49g
Fat:52g
Calories:746
Protein:37g

7.Sheet Pan Roasted Vegetables.

Prep Time:30 mins
Cook Time:1 hr 30 mins
Total Time:2 hrs
Servings:24

Ingredients.
- 8 zucchini, peeled and chopped

- 1 eggplant, peeled and diced
- 8 carrots, diced
- 16 cherry tomatoes
- 2 red onions, sliced
- 1 red bell pepper, sliced
- 1 yellow bell pepper, sliced
- ½ cup olive oil
- 1 teaspoon dried rosemary
- 1 teaspoon dried thyme
- 2 bay leaves, crushed
- 1 teaspoon dried oregano
- 2 cloves garlic, minced
- 2 tablespoons fresh lemon juice
- 1 teaspoon grated lemon zest
- salt and pepper to taste

Directions.

1. Combine zucchini, eggplant, carrots, tomatoes, onions, and peppers in a large bowl. Add oil, rosemary, thyme, bay leaves, oregano, garlic, lemon juice, lemon zest, salt, and pepper. Cover and refrigerate for at least 2 hours, preferably overnight.

2. Preheat the oven to 400°F (200°C).

3. Spread the vegetables on a large roasting pan and roast uncovered for 20 minutes until tomatoes split and some vegetables' edges crisp. Stir and roast for another 20 minutes. Reduce heat to 200°F (95°C) and continue cooking, stirring every 20 minutes, until vegetables are tender.

Nutritional value
Carbs:7g
Fat:5g
Calories:81
Protein:2g

8.Sweet Lentil Soup with Asparagus Tips

Prep Time:15 mins
Cook Time:1 hr 15 mins
Total Time:1 hr 30 mins
Servings:8

Ingredients.
- 3 tablespoons olive oil

- 1 medium head garlic
- ¼ teaspoon dried basil
- 1 red bell pepper
- 2 ½ cups dry lentils
- 2 (32 fluid ounce) containers chicken broth
- 1 ½ large carrot, shredded
- 1 large onion, grated
- 1 cup asparagus tips
- 1 cup sweet peas
- ¼ cup white sugar
- 2 tablespoons orange marmalade
- 2 tablespoons curry powder
- 1 pinch saffron
- 1 teaspoon kosher salt
- ground black pepper to taste

Directions.

1. Preheat your oven to 450 degrees F (230 degrees C).

2. Cut the top off a garlic head and place it in a shallow dish with 2 tablespoons of olive oil and basil. Cover and put on a baking sheet. Halve and seed a bell pepper, drizzle with 1 tablespoon of olive oil, and add to the baking sheet.

3. Bake the garlic and pepper until the pepper browns and the garlic softens, about 20 to 40 minutes. Once cool enough to handle, peel the pepper, chop it, and mash the garlic cloves into a paste.

4. While baking, combine lentils and chicken broth in a large pot over medium heat. Bring to a boil, then simmer for 40 minutes until lentils are tender.

5. Stir in garlic paste, bell pepper, carrots, onion, asparagus, peas, and additional broth if needed. Season with sugar, marmalade, curry powder, saffron, salt, and pepper. Simmer for another 30 minutes until vegetables are tender and flavours meld.

<u>Nutritional value</u>
Carbs:51g
Fat:7g
Calories:319
Protein:17g

9.Garlic Kale Quinoa

Prep Time:10 mins
Cook Time:25 mins

Total Time:35 mins
Servings:2

Ingredients.

- ⅔ cup water
- ⅓ cup quinoa
- 1 tablespoon olive oil
- 1 cup chopped kale
- 1 clove garlic, minced
- salt and ground black pepper to taste
- ¼ teaspoon sesame oil
- 1 tablespoon water, or as needed

Directions.

1. Combine 2/3 cup of water and quinoa in a saucepan. Bring to a boil, then lower the heat to medium-low, cover, and simmer for 15 to 20 minutes until the quinoa is tender and the water is absorbed.

2. In a skillet, heat olive oil over medium heat. Cook kale and garlic in the hot oil until the kale wilts, which should take about 5 minutes. Season with salt and pepper.

3. Mix the cooked quinoa into the kale mixture and add sesame oil. Cook for an additional 5 minutes to blend the flavours. If needed, add 1 tablespoon of water to prevent sticking.

<u>Nutritional value</u>
Carbs:22g
Fat:12g
Calories:188
Protein:5g

Chapter 6: Snacks and Small Bites: Healthy Nibbles

1.Zucchini Yogurt Multigrain Muffins.

Prep Time:15 mins
Cook Time:20 mins
Additional Time:20 mins
Total Time:55 mins
Servings:24

Ingredients.

- 1 ½ cups all-purpose flour
- ¾ cup whole wheat flour
- ¾ cup oat flour
- 1 teaspoon salt
- 1 teaspoon baking soda
- 1 teaspoon baking powder
- 2 ½ teaspoons ground cinnamon
- ¼ teaspoon ground nutmeg
- 3 eggs
- ½ cup vegetable oil

Directions.

1. Preheat your oven to 400°F (200°C) and lightly grease 24 muffin cups.

2. In one bowl, combine all-purpose flour, whole wheat flour, oat flour, salt, baking powder, baking soda, cinnamon, and nutmeg. In another bowl, whisk together eggs, vegetable oil, applesauce, yogurt, sugar, honey, and vanilla extract. Gradually add the flour mixture to the egg mixture, stirring until just combined. Gently fold in the grated zucchini, carrots, pecans, and raisins. Spoon the batter into the prepared muffin cups.

3. Bake for 18 to 20 minutes in the preheated oven, or until a toothpick inserted into the centre of a muffin comes out clean. Allow the muffins to cool in the pan for 10 minutes before transferring them to wire racks to cool completely.

Nutritional value
Carbs:33g
Fat:8g
Calories:207
Protein:4g

2.Applesauce Cake

Prep Time:15 mins
Cook Time:40 mins
Total Time:55 mins
Servings:12

Ingredients.

- 1 cup white sugar
- ½ cup butter
- 1 cup chilled applesauce
- 2 cups all-purpose flour
- 1 teaspoon baking soda
- 1 teaspoon ground cinnamon
- ¼ teaspoon ground cloves
- ½ cup chopped walnuts
- ½ cup raisins

Directions.

1. Gather all your ingredients. Preheat your oven to
350°F (175°C). Grease and flour an 8-inch cake pan.

2. Use an electric mixer to beat together the sugar and butter in a large bowl until creamy. Add the applesauce and beat well.

3. Stir in the flour, baking soda, cinnamon, and cloves until just mixed.

4. Gently fold in the walnuts and raisins.

5. Spoon the cake batter into the prepared pan.

6. Bake in the preheated oven until a toothpick inserted into the centre comes out clean, which should take about 40 minutes.

7. Serve the cake warm and enjoy!

<u>Nutritional value</u>
Carbs:41g
Fat:14g
Calories:271
Protein:3g

3.Creamy Cottage Cheese Scrambled Eggs

Prep Time:5 mins

Cook Time:5 mins
Total Time:10 mins
Servings:2

Ingredients.

- 1 tablespoon butter
- 4 large eggs, beaten
- ¼ cup cottage cheese
- 1 teaspoon chopped fresh chives, or to taste (Optional)
- ground black pepper to taste

Directions.

1. Prepare all the necessary ingredients.

2. Heat butter in a skillet over medium heat. Pour in beaten eggs and allow them to cook without stirring until the edges start to set, which usually takes 1 to 2 minutes.

3. Mix cottage cheese and chives into the eggs, and season with black pepper.

4. Continue cooking and stirring until the eggs are almost fully set, about 3 to 4 minutes more.

<u>**Nutritional value**</u>
Carbs:2g
Fat:17g
Calories:224
Protein:16g

4.Seattle Smoked Salmon Dip

Prep Time:10 mins
Additional Time:1 hr
Total Time:1 hr 10 mins
Servings:20

Ingredients.

- 4 ounces flaked smoked salmon, skin and bones removed
- 1 (8 ounce) package cream cheese, softened
- 1 cup shredded white Cheddar cheese, divided
- ½ cup mayonnaise
- 2 tablespoons chopped green onions
- 2 tablespoons milk
- 1 tablespoon lemon juice

- 1 (1 ounce) package McCormick® Guacamole Seasoning Mix

Directions.

1. Combine all ingredients thoroughly in a large bowl. Cover the mixture.
2. Chill in the refrigerator for 1 hour or until you're ready to serve. Optionally, decorate with extra green onions before serving.

<u>Nutritional value</u>
Carbs:2g
Fat:10g
Calories:115
Protein:3g

5.Raspberry Nut Butter Cake

Servings:14

Ingredients.
- 6 eggs
- 1 cup butter, softened

- 1 ½ cups white sugar
- ¾ cup seedless raspberry jam
- 1 tablespoon vanilla extract
- ¼ cup dark rum
- 1 cup all-purpose flour
- 1 teaspoon baking powder
- ¾ cup ground walnuts
- ¾ cup ground pecans

Directions.

1. Preheat your oven to 350 degrees Fahrenheit (175 degrees Celsius) and prepare a 9-inch tube pan by greasing and flouring it.

2. Separate the eggs. In a bowl, whisk the egg whites until they form stiff peaks. Set them aside.

3. In a large bowl, cream together the butter and sugar until smooth. Mix in the egg yolks, followed by the jam, vanilla extract, and dark rum.

4. In another bowl, combine the flour and baking powder. Gradually add this mixture to the creamed mixture, then stir in the nuts. Fold about a third of the beaten egg whites into the batter to lighten it, then gently fold in the remaining egg whites until

fully incorporated. Pour the batter into the prepared pan.

5. Bake at 350 degrees F (175 degrees C) for 65 to 70 minutes, or until a toothpick inserted near the centre comes out clean. Allow the cake to cool on a rack. This recipe yields about 12 servings.

Nutritional value
Carbs:42g
Fat:21g
Calories:380
Protein:5g

6.Carrot Zucchini Bread

Prep Time:30 mins
Cook Time:1 hr 20 mins
Additional Time:2 hrs
Total Time:3 hrs 50 mins
Servings:16

Ingredients.

- 1 cup all-purpose flour
- 1 ½ cups whole wheat flour
- 1 teaspoon baking soda

- ¼ teaspoon baking powder
- 1 tablespoon ground cinnamon
- 1 teaspoon ground nutmeg
- ½ teaspoon ground cloves
- 1 teaspoon salt
- 6 egg whites
- ½ cup unsweetened applesauce
- 1 ½ cups brown sugar
- 1 cup grated unpeeled zucchini
- 1 cup grated carrot
- 2 teaspoons vanilla extract
- ½ cup raisins
- ½ cup chopped pecans

Directions.

1. Preheat your oven to 325 degrees Fahrenheit (165 degrees Celsius) and grease a 9x5 inch loaf pan with non-stick spray. In a large bowl, sift together all-purpose flour, whole wheat flour, baking soda, baking powder, cinnamon, nutmeg, cloves, and salt until evenly mixed.

2. Using a mixer, beat the egg whites until they are light and frothy. Stir in applesauce, brown sugar, grated zucchini, grated carrots, and vanilla extract

until thoroughly combined. Add the raisins and pecans, mixing well. Gradually add the flour mixture, stirring until just blended. Pour the batter into the greased loaf pan.

3. Bake for approximately 1 hour and 20 minutes, or until a toothpick inserted into the centre comes out clean. Let the bread cool in the pan for 10 minutes before removing it and allowing it to cool completely on a wire rack.

Nutritional value
Carbs:35g
Fat:3g
Calories:173
Protein:4g

7.Steamed Squash Medley with Sun-Dried Tomatoes

Prep Time:15 mins
Cook Time:15 mins
Additional Time:10 mins
Total Time:40 mins
Servings:6

Ingredients.

- 6 dehydrated sun-dried tomatoes
- 2 cups boiling water
- 6 small zucchini, sliced
- 6 small yellow squash, sliced
- 1 sweet onion, chopped
- 2 tablespoons butter
- 1 teaspoon white sugar
- ¼ teaspoon freshly ground black pepper
- salt to taste

Directions.

1. Place sun-dried tomatoes in a bowl with boiling water and let them soak for 10 minutes. Remove tomatoes with a slotted spoon, chop them coarsely, and keep the water.

2. Pour the reserved sun-dried tomato water into a saucepan and bring it to a boil. Place chopped sun-dried tomatoes, zucchini, squash, and onion in a steamer basket over the boiling water. Reduce heat to low, cover, and simmer for 15 minutes or until vegetables are tender. Discard the water.

3. Transfer steamed vegetables to a bowl and mix with butter, sugar, pepper, and salt before serving.

<u>**Nutritional value**</u>
Carbs:15g
Fat:5g
Calories:105
Protein:6g

Chapter 7: Desserts and Beverages: Indulgence with Care

1.White Peach Sorbet:

Prep Time:30 mins
Additional Time:1 hr
Total Time:1 hr 30 mins
Servings:6

Ingredients.
- 5 ripe white peaches
- 2 teaspoons lemon juice
- 2 teaspoons white sugar, or to taste

Directions.

1. Peel white peaches, leaving some skin for texture and colour. Cut the peach flesh into chunks,

discard the pits, and place the chunks in a bowl. Add lemon juice.

2. Use an immersion blender to puree the peaches and lemon juice until smooth. Stir in sugar to your liking, then blend again. Refrigerate the peach mixture for 1 hour to chill.

3. Transfer the chilled peach mixture into an ice cream maker and freeze following the manufacturer's instructions.

Nutritional value
Carbs:9g
Fat:0
Calories:38
Protein:1g

2.Pineapple Upside-Down Cake.

Prep Time:20 mins
Cook Time:30 mins
Additional Time:10 mins
Total Time:1 hr
Servings:12

Ingredients.

- 1 (20 ounce) can pineapple rings
- ¼ cup water, or as needed
- ½ cup unsalted butter
- 1 (15.25 ounce) package white cake mix (such as Betty Crocker Super Moist)
- ½ cup vegetable oil
- 3 large egg whites
- 1 ½ cups brown sugar
- 7 maraschino cherries

Directions.

1. Preheat your oven to 350 degrees Fahrenheit (175 degrees Celsius).

2. Drain the liquid from canned pineapple into a 1-cup measuring cup. If needed, add water to reach 1 cup. Keep 7 pineapple rings and the juice aside for the cake, saving any extra for later use.

3. Heat butter in a 10- or 11-inch cast iron skillet over medium-high heat.

4. While the butter melts, mix together the cake mix, the reserved 1 cup of pineapple juice, vegetable oil, and egg whites in a bowl. Beat with an electric mixer on medium speed for 2 minutes.

5. Take the melted butter off the heat and evenly sprinkle brown sugar over it until covered. Arrange 6 pineapple rings around the skillet's edge and place the remaining ring in the centre, ensuring they do not overlap. Put a maraschino cherry in the centre of each pineapple ring. Pour the cake batter over the pineapples.

6. Bake in the preheated oven for about 30-35 minutes or until a toothpick inserted in the centre comes out clean.

7. Remove from the oven and let it cool in the skillet for 10 minutes. Be careful not to let the cake cool too much as it may stick to the pan.

8. Run an offset spatula around the edges to loosen the cake. Place a plate over the skillet, then carefully flip and turn out the warm cake onto the plate. Transfer any fruit or glaze left in the skillet back onto the cake.

Nutritional value
Carbs:59g
Fat:18g
Calories:401

Protein:3g

3.Greek Yogurt Chia Pudding

Prep Time:10 mins
RefrigeratedTime:8 hrs
Total Time:8 hrs 10 mins
Servings:2 servings

Ingredients.
- 1 (5.3 ounce) container vanilla Greek yoghourt
- 2/3 cup milk
- 2 tablespoons chia seeds
- 1/2 tablespoon honey, or more to taste
- 1 cup chopped fresh fruit

Directions.
1. Combine Greek yoghurt, milk, chia seeds, and honey in a small bowl, mixing thoroughly.
2. Cover the bowl and refrigerate overnight.
3. Stir the mixture before serving to evenly distribute any settled seeds. Add your preferred fruit on top and enjoy!

<u>**Nutritional value**</u>
Carbs:33g
Fat:7g
Calories:237
Protein:12g

4.Ginger-Turmeric Herbal Tea

Prep Time:5 mins
Cook Time:15 mins
Total Time:20 mins
Servings:2

Ingredients.

- 2 cups water
- ½ teaspoon ground turmeric
- ½ teaspoon chopped fresh ginger
- ½ teaspoon ground cinnamon
- 1 tablespoon honey
- 1 lemon wedge

Directions.

1. Collect all the necessary ingredients.

2. Boil water in a small saucepan, then add turmeric, ginger, and cinnamon.

3. Lower the heat and let it simmer for 10 minutes.

4. Pour the tea through a strainer into a large glass.

5. Mix in honey and serve with a wedge of lemon.

Nutritional value
Carbs:10g
Fat:0
Calories:37
Protein:0

5.Coffee Gelatin Dessert

Prep Time:10 mins
Cook Time:5 mins
Additional Time:6 hrs
Total Time:6 hrs 15 mins
Servings:5

Ingredients.

- ¾ cup white sugar
- 3 (.25 ounce) envelopes unflavored gelatin powder
- 3 cups hot brewed coffee

- 1 ⅓ cups water
- 1 tablespoon lemon juice
- 1 cup sweetened whipped cream for garnish

Directions.

1. Combine sugar and gelatin in a saucepan. Add hot coffee and water. Heat gently, stirring often until sugar and gelatin dissolve completely. Remove from heat, mix in lemon juice. Pour into a 4 1/2 cup mould. Chill until firm, at least 6 hours or overnight. Serve with whipped cream.

Nutritional value
Carbs:32g
Fat:12g
Calories:215
Protein:6g

BONUS

30-Day Meal Plan.

Week 1

Day 1:

Breakfast: Oatmeal with fresh berries and a drizzle of honey.
Lunch: Grilled chicken salad with mixed greens, cucumbers, tomatoes, and a light vinaigrette.
Dinner: Baked salmon with steamed broccoli and quinoa.
Snack: Apple slices with almond butter.

Day 2:

*Breakfast:*Greek yoghourt with granola and sliced bananas.

*Lunch:*Turkey and avocado wrap with whole grain tortilla.

Dinner: Stir-fried tofu with mixed vegetables and brown rice.

*Snack:*Carrot sticks with hummus.

Day 3:

Breakfast: Smoothie with spinach, banana, and almond milk.

Lunch: Lentil soup with a side of whole grain bread.

Dinner: Grilled shrimp with a side of sweet potato and asparagus.

Snack: Handful of mixed nuts.

Day 4:

Breakfast: Scrambled eggs with spinach and whole grain toast.

Lunch: Quinoa salad with chickpeas, cherry tomatoes, and feta cheese.

Dinner: Baked chicken breast with roasted Brussels sprouts and mashed cauliflower.
Snack: Fresh berries.

Day 5:
Breakfast: Whole grain pancakes with a side of mixed fruit.
Lunch: Spinach and mushroom omelette with a side salad.
Dinner: Baked cod with a side of sautéed green beans and wild rice.
Snack: Cottage cheese with pineapple chunks.

Day 6:
Breakfast: Chia seed pudding with mixed berries.
Lunch: Grilled vegetable wrap with hummus.
Dinner: Turkey meatballs with zucchini noodles and marinara sauce.
Snack: Sliced cucumber with tzatziki.

Day 7:
Breakfast: Smoothie bowl with mixed fruits, granola, and chia seeds.

Lunch: Chicken and vegetable soup with a side of whole grain crackers.

Dinner: Stuffed bell peppers with ground turkey, quinoa, and vegetables.

Snack: Pear slices with a few walnuts.

Week 2

Day 8:

Breakfast: Overnight oats with chia seeds and strawberries.

Lunch: Tuna salad on whole grain bread with a side of mixed greens.

Dinner: Lemon garlic shrimp with quinoa and steamed spinach.

Snack: Sliced bell peppers with guacamole.

Day 9:

*Breakfast:*Smoothie with kale, pineapple, and coconut water.

Lunch: Lentil and vegetable stew with a side of whole grain roll.

Dinner: Baked chicken thighs with roasted sweet potatoes and sautéed kale.

Snack: Dried apricots with a few almonds.

Day 10:

Breakfast: Greek yoghourt parfait with granola and blueberries.

Lunch: Spinach and strawberry salad with grilled chicken and balsamic dressing.

Dinner: Broiled tilapia with a side of quinoa and roasted Brussels sprouts.

Snack: Apple slices with a handful of raisins.

Day 11:

Breakfast: Whole grain cereal with almond milk and sliced bananas.

Lunch: Turkey and avocado salad with mixed greens and a light lemon dressing.

Dinner: Grilled lamb chops with a side of roasted carrots and brown rice.

Snack: Fresh mango slices.

Day 12:

Breakfast: Smoothie with spinach, mango, and flaxseeds.

Lunch: Chickpea and vegetable curry with a side of brown rice.

*Dinner:*Baked pork tenderloin with roasted Brussels sprouts and mashed sweet potatoes.

Snack: Greek yoghourt with a drizzle of honey.

Day 13:

Breakfast: Oatmeal with almond butter and sliced apples.

Lunch: Quinoa and black bean salad with avocado and lime dressing.

Dinner: Grilled salmon with a side of asparagus and wild rice.

Snack: Celery sticks with peanut butter.

Day 14:

Breakfast: Smoothie bowl with spinach, berries, and granola.

Lunch: Lentil and vegetable soup with a side of whole grain bread.

Dinner: Baked chicken breast with a side of roasted sweet potatoes and green beans.

Snack: Sliced oranges.

Week 3

Day 15:
Breakfast: Whole grain toast with avocado and poached egg.
Lunch: Turkey wrap with spinach, avocado, and whole grain tortilla.
Dinner: Baked cod with a side of quinoa and sautéed kale.
Snack: Mixed berry medley.

Day 16:
Breakfast: Greek yoghourt with sliced peaches and granola.
Lunch: Mixed greens salad with chickpeas, cucumbers, and a light lemon dressing.
*Dinner:*Grilled shrimp with a side of steamed broccoli and brown rice.
Snack: Sliced cucumber with hummus.

Day 17:

Breakfast: Smoothie with kale, banana, and almond milk.

Lunch: Spinach and mushroom omelette with a side salad.

Dinner: Baked chicken thighs with roasted carrots and wild rice.

Snack: Sliced apple with almond butter.

Day 18:

Breakfast: Oatmeal with fresh blueberries and a drizzle of honey.

Lunch: Quinoa and black bean salad with avocado and lime dressing.

Dinner: Broiled tilapia with a side of steamed asparagus and mashed sweet potatoes.

Snack: Mixed nuts.

Day 19:

Breakfast: Chia seed pudding with mixed berries.

Lunch: Tuna salad with mixed greens and whole grain crackers.

Dinner: Grilled turkey burgers with a side of roasted sweet potatoes and green beans.

Snack: Fresh pineapple chunks.

Day 20:

Breakfast: Smoothie bowl with spinach, pineapple, and granola.

*Lunch:*Chicken and vegetable soup with a side of whole grain roll.

Dinner: Baked salmon with a side of quinoa and roasted Brussels sprouts.

Snack: Sliced bell peppers with guacamole.

Day 21:

Breakfast: Whole grain pancakes with a side of mixed fruit.

Lunch: Spinach and strawberry salad with grilled chicken and balsamic dressing.

Dinner: Stuffed bell peppers with ground turkey, quinoa, and vegetables.

Snack: Carrot sticks with hummus.

Week 4

Day 22:

Breakfast: Greek yoghourt parfait with granola and sliced bananas.

Lunch: Turkey and avocado wrap with whole grain tortilla.

Dinner: Lemon garlic shrimp with brown rice and steamed broccoli.

Snack: Sliced apples with almond butter.

Day 23:

Breakfast: Smoothie with kale, pineapple, and coconut water.

Lunch: Lentil and vegetable stew with a side of whole grain roll.

Dinner: Baked chicken thighs with roasted Brussels sprouts and mashed cauliflower.

Snack:Fresh mango slices.

Day 24:

Breakfast: Oatmeal with sliced apples and cinnamon.

Lunch: Spinach and mushroom omelette with a side salad.

Dinner: Baked cod with a side of wild rice and steamed asparagus.

Snack: Celery sticks with peanut butter.

Day 25:

Breakfast: Smoothie with spinach, banana, and almond milk.

*Lunch:*Quinoa salad with chickpeas, cherry tomatoes, and feta cheese.

Dinner: Baked pork tenderloin with roasted carrots and green beans.

Snack: Greek yoghourt with a drizzle of honey.

Day 26:

Breakfast: Whole grain cereal with almond milk and sliced strawberries.

Lunch: Turkey and avocado salad with mixed greens and a light lemon dressing.

Dinner: Baked chicken breast with a side of roasted sweet potatoes and steamed broccoli.

Snack: Sliced bell peppers with guacamole.

Day 27:

Breakfast: Smoothie bowl with spinach, mixed berries, and granola.

Lunch: Lentil and vegetable soup with a side of whole grain bread.

Dinner: Grilled lamb chops with a side of roasted Brussels sprouts and quinoa.
Snack: Mixed berry medley.

Day 28:

Breakfast: Whole grain toast with avocado and scrambled eggs.
Lunch: Grilled vegetable wrap with hummus.
Dinner: Baked salmon with a side of wild rice and steamed spinach.
Snack: Fresh pineapple chunks.

Day 29:

Breakfast: Greek yoghourts with granola and blueberries.
Lunch: Spinach and strawberry salad with grilled chicken and balsamic dressing.
Dinner: Broiled tilapia with a side of quinoa and roasted Brussels sprouts.
Snack: Apple slices with a handful of walnuts.

Day 30:

Breakfast: Smoothie with kale, mango, and almond milk.

Lunch: Chickpea and vegetable curry with a side of brown rice.

Dinner: Baked chicken breast with roasted sweet potatoes and sautéed green beans.

Snack: Fresh berries.

30-Day Meal Plan Journal.

WEEKLY MEAL PLAN JOURNAL

WEEK OF: _______

SUN	BREAKFAST:	DINNER:
	LUNCH:	SNACK:
MON	BREAKFAST:	DINNER:
	LUNCH:	SNACK:
TUE	BREAKFAST:	DINNER:
	LUNCH:	SNACK:
WED	BREAKFAST:	DINNER:
	LUNCH:	SNACK:
THU	BREAKFAST:	DINNER:
	LUNCH:	SNACK:
FRI	BREAKFAST:	DINNER:
	LUNCH:	SNACK:
SAT	BREAKFAST:	DINNER:
	LUNCH:	SNACK:

WEEKLY MEAL PLAN JOURNAL

WEEK OF: _________

SUN	BREAKFAST:	DINNER:
	LUNCH:	SNACK:
MON	BREAKFAST:	DINNER:
	LUNCH:	SNACK:
TUE	BREAKFAST:	DINNER:
	LUNCH:	SNACK:
WED	BREAKFAST:	DINNER:
	LUNCH:	SNACK:
THU	BREAKFAST:	DINNER:
	LUNCH:	SNACK:
FRI	BREAKFAST:	DINNER:
	LUNCH:	SNACK:
SAT	BREAKFAST:	DINNER:
	LUNCH:	SNACK:

WEEKLY MEAL PLAN JOURNAL

WEEK OF: _________

SUN	BREAKFAST:	DINNER:
	LUNCH:	SNACK:
MON	BREAKFAST:	DINNER:
	LUNCH:	SNACK:
TUE	BREAKFAST:	DINNER:
	LUNCH:	SNACK:
WED	BREAKFAST:	DINNER:
	LUNCH:	SNACK:
THU	BREAKFAST:	DINNER:
	LUNCH:	SNACK:
FRI	BREAKFAST:	DINNER:
	LUNCH:	SNACK:
SAT	BREAKFAST:	DINNER:
	LUNCH:	SNACK:

WEEKLY MEAL PLAN JOURNAL

WEEK OF: __________

SUN	BREAKFAST:	DINNER:
	LUNCH:	SNACK:
MON	BREAKFAST:	DINNER:
	LUNCH:	SNACK:
TUE	BREAKFAST:	DINNER:
	LUNCH:	SNACK:
WED	BREAKFAST:	DINNER:
	LUNCH:	SNACK:
THU	BREAKFAST:	DINNER:
	LUNCH:	SNACK:
FRI	BREAKFAST:	DINNER:
	LUNCH:	SNACK:
SAT	BREAKFAST:	DINNER:
	LUNCH:	SNACK:

Food list Encyclopaedia

1.Citrus Fruits

Oranges, Grapefruits, Lemons, and Limes: These fruits are packed with vitamin C, essential for a robust immune system. Vitamin C helps increase the production of white blood cells, which fight infections.

2.Berries

Blueberries, Strawberries, and Raspberries: Berries are high in antioxidants, particularly vitamin C and flavonoids, which help protect cells from damage and support immune health.

3.Leafy Greens

Spinach, Kale, and Swiss Chard: These greens are rich in vitamins A, C, and E, as well as fibre and antioxidants. They enhance immune function and can be easily added to soups, salads, and smoothies.

4.Garlic

Fresh Garlic Cloves: Garlic has been used for its medicinal properties for centuries. It boosts the immune system thanks to its sulphur-containing compounds, like allicin, which have potent antimicrobial effects.

5.Ginger

Fresh Ginger Root: Ginger helps reduce inflammation and nausea, and its antioxidant properties can strengthen the immune response. It can be added to teas, smoothies, or as a spice in cooking.

6.Turmeric

Ground Turmeric Powder: Turmeric contains curcumin, a compound with powerful anti-inflammatory and antioxidant properties. It's great in curries, soups, and can even be added to your morning smoothie.

Foods Rich in Nutrients and Hydration

1.Bone Broth

Chicken or Beef Broth: Bone broth is rich in vitamins and minerals, including collagen, which supports gut health. It's easy to digest and provides hydration, making it ideal for recovery from illnesses like ehrlichiosis.

2.Coconut Water

Natural Coconut Water: This drink is a fantastic source of electrolytes and hydration, important for maintaining energy levels and supporting cellular function during illness.

3.Herbal Teas

Chamomile, Peppermint, and Echinacea Teas: These teas not only provide warmth and comfort but also have various healing properties. Echinacea, for instance, is known for its immune-boosting effects.

Protein-Packed Foods

1.Lean Meats

Chicken Breast and Turkey: These meats are high in protein, necessary for tissue repair and immune function. They also contain zinc, a mineral that helps in the production of immune cells.

2. Fish

Salmon, Tuna, and Mackerel: Rich in omega-3 fatty acids, these fish have anti-inflammatory properties and support overall immune health. They're also an excellent source of protein.

3. Legumes

Lentils, Chickpeas, and Beans: These are packed with protein, fibre, and essential vitamins and minerals, making them a staple for a balanced diet and sustained energy.

Foods That Help Fight Fatigue

1. Whole Grains

Oats, Quinoa, and Brown Rice: These grains are high in fibre and complex carbohydrates, providing long-lasting energy and stabilising blood sugar levels.

2.Nuts and Seeds

Almonds, Walnuts, and Chia Seeds: These are nutrient-dense and provide a quick energy boost. They are rich in healthy fats, proteins, and antioxidants.

3.Dark Chocolate

70% Cocoa or Higher: Dark chocolate is not only delicious but also a great source of antioxidants. It can help improve brain function and provide a small energy boost.

Foods to Avoid

1.Processed Foods
Packaged Snacks and Ready-to-Eat Meals: These often contain high levels of sugar, salt, and unhealthy fats, which can weaken the immune system and increase inflammation.

2.Sugary Beverages

Sodas and Energy Drinks: These drinks can cause blood sugar spikes and contribute to inflammation. Opt for water or herbal teas instead.

3.Alcohol

Beer, Wine, and Spirits: Alcohol can suppress the immune system and dehydrate the body, making it harder to fight off infections like ehrlichiosis.

SMART SHOPPERS GUIDE TO DECODING FOOD LABEL

Here's how you can become a smart shopper by decoding food labels and making choices that support your health and safety.

Why Food Labels Matter

Food labels are like the book covers of what we eat—they give us a snapshot of what's inside. Knowing how to read these labels is vital, especially for those with health conditions like ehrlichiosis, which can weaken the immune system and make you more susceptible to other illnesses. By choosing foods wisely, you can boost your immune system and reduce the risk of complications.

Key Elements of Food Labels

1.Ingredients List

The ingredients list is where you start. Ingredients are listed in order of quantity, from highest to lowest. Look for simple, whole foods at the top of the list. If you see a lot of long, hard-to-pronounce names, it might be a sign that the product is heavily processed.

2.Nutrition Facts

This section breaks down the nutritional content of the food. Pay attention to calories, fats, sodium, and sugars. For someone dealing with ehrlichiosis, a balanced diet with minimal processed sugars and fats can help maintain a strong immune system.

3.Serving Size

Always check the serving size. Manufacturers often list nutritional information based on a serving that's smaller than what you might actually eat. Understanding serving sizes helps you accurately assess the amount of nutrients and calories you're consuming.

4. Expiration Date

Foods past their expiration dates can lose nutritional value and may become unsafe to eat. This is particularly important for those with weakened immune systems. Always choose fresh products and avoid anything close to its expiration date.

5.Allergens

Even if you don't have known allergies, knowing common allergens is crucial. Food allergies can sometimes flare up unexpectedly, especially when your immune system is compromised by illnesses like ehrlichiosis. Check for common allergens like nuts, dairy, and gluten.

What to Look For

1.Whole Foods

Opt for foods that are as close to their natural state as possible. Fresh fruits, vegetables, lean proteins, and whole grains are your best bets. These foods provide essential nutrients that support your body's defences.

2.Organic and Non-GMO Labels

Organic foods are grown without synthetic pesticides or fertilisers, which is beneficial for overall health. Non-GMO labels indicate that the food hasn't been genetically modified. While there's debate about GMOs, choosing organic can reduce your exposure to potentially harmful substances.

3.Low-Sodium and Low-Sugar Options

Excess sodium and sugar can strain your body, especially if it's fighting off infections. Look for labels that highlight "low sodium" or "no added sugars." This can help keep your immune system in good shape.

4.Fortified Foods

Some foods are fortified with vitamins and minerals. These can be particularly useful if your diet is lacking in certain nutrients. For example, vitamin D and zinc are important for immune health.

5.Antibiotic-Free and Hormone-Free Meats

Choosing meats that are free from antibiotics and hormones is important. These additives can affect your health, especially if your body is already dealing with an illness. Look for labels that certify the meat as "antibiotic-free" or "hormone-free."

Be Cautious of Marketing Tricks

Natural: This term isn't regulated and can be misleading. It doesn't necessarily mean the food is healthy or free from chemicals.

Light: Often refers to flavour or colour rather than a reduction in calories or fat.

Reduced-Fat: Might have less fat but could be higher in sugar to make up for the taste.

Building a Healthy Shopping List

Vegetables and Fruits: Fresh, frozen, or canned without added sugars or sodium.

Lean Proteins: Chicken, turkey, fish, eggs, and legumes.

Whole Grains: Brown rice, quinoa, whole-wheat pasta, and oats.

Dairy or Dairy Alternatives: Low-fat or non-dairy options like almond milk or yoghurt.

Healthy Fats: Olive oil, avocados, nuts, and seeds.

www.ingramcontent.com/pod-product-compliance
Lightning Source LLC
Chambersburg PA
CBHW071024250726
48653CB00005B/1698